DISCOVER THE SECRET OF THE HOLLYWOOD DIET

Unlock the Secret of How Movie Stars Enjoy Rapid Weight Loss, Body Detoxification, with Quick and Easy Grapefruit Diet Recipes

CAROLINE SIMMONS, MD

Copyright Page

Copyright © 2024 by Caroline Simmons, MD.

All rights reserved. No part of this book may be reproduced, stored in a retrieval system, or transmitted in any form or by any means, electronic, mechanical, photocopying, recording, or otherwise, without the prior written permission of the author, except in the case of brief quotations embodied in critical articles and reviews.

The recipes and suggestions provided in this book are for informational purposes only. The author and publisher are not responsible for any adverse effects or consequences resulting from the use of the recipes, dietary practices, or suggestions described herein. Always consult a professional or medical expert if you have any concerns regarding your dietary needs and health conditions.

Table of Contents

INTRODUCTION

Nearly 25 years ago, in 1997, the original Hollywood 48-Hour Miracle Diet was introduced with a simple yet ambitious goal: to help people lose weight quickly. This unique juice blend is packed with essential vitamins and minerals, along with carefully chosen essential oils, to ensure that your body stays balanced while you take a break from food for two days.

The Hollywood 48-Hour Miracle Diet isn't just another fad; it's a carefully crafted program designed to give your body a reset. By combining a powerful mix of nutrients, this juice supports your body's natural functions, keeping you energized and healthy even as you fast. It's a versatile option that fits into busy lifestyles, providing a quick and effective way to jumpstart weight loss and refresh your system.

Whether you're looking to shed a few pounds before a big event, kick off a longer-term weight loss journey, or simply give your body a much-needed detox, the Hollywood 48-Hour Miracle Diet offers a convenient and effective solution. It's about more than just losing weight—it's about feeling rejuvenated, balanced, and ready to take on whatever comes next.

1

WHAT EXACTLY IS THE HOLLYWOOD DIET?

The Hollywood Diet is all about helping you lose weight without sacrificing the nutrients your body needs to feel its best. These tasty, low-calorie drinks are designed to help you shed those extra pounds, reset your body's chemistry, and feel more confident in your own skin.

The great thing about The Hollywood Diet is that it works fast. The 24-Hour Miracle Diet and the 48-

Hour Miracle Diet are specifically made to give you noticeable results in just a day or two, not weeks. This isn't like those fad diets that pop up every few years and then disappear. The Hollywood Diet has been around for a long time and has scientific studies backing up its effectiveness. People have reported losing anywhere from 2 to 16.5 pounds in just 24 to 48 hours by following the plan as directed.

What sets The Hollywood Diet apart is that you get these quick results without feeling drained and sluggish, which often happens with crash diets. Plus, unlike other juice cleanses or liquid diets, most people don't experience uncomfortable digestive issues like cramping or stomach pain.

The Hollywood Diet has proven to be a reliable way to achieve quick weight loss while still keeping your health in check. With its long history of success and many positive reviews, it's a great option for anyone looking to kickstart their weight loss journey quickly and effectively.

Why Do Celebrities Love the Hollywood Diet?

Fast Results:

One of the main attractions is how quickly it works. The 24-Hour Miracle Diet and the 48-Hour Miracle Diet promise noticeable weight loss in just a day or two. This is perfect for stars who need to look their best for last-minute events or photoshoots.

Easy and Convenient:

With their packed schedules, celebrities need something that fits seamlessly into their lives. The Hollywood Diet drinks are ready-to-go, making it super easy to follow without any complicated meal prep or planning.

Keeps You Healthy:

Even though it's a low-calorie diet, The Hollywood Dict provides essential nutrients. This means celebrities can lose weight while still feeling energetic and healthy, which is crucial given their busy and demanding lives.

Trusted and Proven:

The Hollywood Diet has been around for a long time and has a lot of positive reviews and scientific backing. Celebrities trust it because they know it works and don't have to worry about trying something unproven.

No Bad Side Effects:

Many quick diets leave people feeling tired or with digestive issues. The Hollywood Diet is known for delivering fast results without these problems, so celebrities can keep up with their hectic schedules without feeling sluggish.

Celebrity Endorsements:

Word spreads quickly in Hollywood. Many stars have tried and loved The Hollywood Diet, and they share their success stories with their peers, leading more celebrities to give it a try.

Media Coverage:

The Hollywood Diet gets a lot of media attention, so it's well-known among celebrities who keep up with trends and want to stay in shape.

In short, celebrities love The Hollywood Diet because it offers quick, reliable results, is easy to use, keeps them healthy, and has a proven track record. It fits perfectly into their busy lives, helping them look and feel great on and off the red carpet.

Understanding the Hollywood Diet

The Hollywood diet is often talked about as a quick way to lose weight and achieve a slimmer figure, much like the transformations we see on the big screen. But what exactly is this diet, and why do so many people, including celebrities, turn to it?

At its heart, the Hollywood diet is about rapid weight loss. Many versions of this diet promise to help you shed pounds quickly by drastically cutting calories. This can mean replacing regular meals with things like juices, shakes, or special diet cookies. The idea is to get fast results, which is especially appealing if you have a special event coming up or just want to see a quick change.

However, while the promise of losing weight fast is tempting, it's important to approach the Hollywood diet with caution. Cutting calories too drastically can lead to short-term weight loss, but it also comes with some downsides. You might lose muscle along with fat, feel tired and weak, and miss out on important nutrients your body needs. Plus, these diets are hard to stick with for a long time, so the weight often comes back once you start eating normally again.

Still, many people are drawn to the Hollywood diet because it offers a quick fix. If you're considering it, think of it as a temporary measure rather than a permanent solution. It's always a good idea to talk to a healthcare professional before starting any drastic diet to make sure it's safe for you.

Remember, while the idea of rapid weight loss can be appealing, making gradual changes to your eating and exercise habits is usually a healthier and more effective approach in the long run. The Hollywood diet reflects our fascination with celebrity culture and the desire for quick results, but true, lasting change comes from adopting sustainable, healthy habits.

So, if you're inspired by the Hollywood diet, use it as a stepping stone to kickstart your journey, but focus on building a lifestyle that supports your overall well-being for the long haul.

2

THE ORIGINS OF THE HOLLYWOOD DIET

The origins of the Hollywood Diet are as fascinating as the stars who made it famous. Picture Hollywood in the 1980s: a world where looking good was everything and the pressure to stay slim was intense. In this high-stakes environment, a new diet began making waves—a juice cleanse that promised quick and dramatic weight loss.

The Hollywood Diet started as a simple idea: replace your meals with a special blend of fruit juices for a day or two, and watch the pounds melt away. It was the perfect solution for actors and actresses who needed to lose weight fast for a movie role or a red carpet event. The appeal was immediate results, something that was incredibly attractive in a world where looking perfect was part of the job.

Word spread quickly among the Hollywood elite, and soon celebrities were endorsing this diet, sharing their success stories and boosting its popularity. The idea that you could lose up to 10 pounds in just 48 hours seemed almost magical, and before long, the Hollywood Diet became a household name. It wasn't just a diet; it was a secret weapon for anyone looking to make a quick transformation.

Over the years, the Hollywood Diet has changed a bit, with new versions and tweaks, but the basic concept remains the same: a fast, effective way to shed weight and feel great. It's not a long-term solution, but for many, it's the quick fix they need to feel confident and camera-ready.

At its heart, the Hollywood Diet is a reflection of the unique pressures of life in the limelight. It shows the lengths to which people will go to achieve their ideal image and the constant quest for quick fixes in the world of health and beauty. While it may not be for everyone, its origins and lasting popularity speak volumes about the ongoing desire for rapid results and the influence of Hollywood glamour on our everyday lives.

Understanding the Core Concepts of the Hollywood Diet

The Hollywood Diet has gained popularity thanks to its promise of quick weight loss, often endorsed by celebrities. Let's break down its key principles in a way that's relatable and easy to understand.

1. Calorie Restriction

The main idea behind the Hollywood Diet is to eat fewer calories than your body needs, creating a calorie deficit that leads to weight loss. Typically, this diet limits your intake to about 800-1200 calories a day. While this can help you lose weight fast, it's important to be careful and ensure you still get the nutrients your body needs.

2. Short-Term Focus

This diet isn't meant to be a long-term solution. It usually lasts from one day to a few days, providing a quick fix for those looking to shed pounds rapidly. Think of it as a way to jump-start your weight loss or to slim down quickly for a special event.

3. Pre-Planned Meals

The Hollywood Diet often includes specific meal plans or pre-packaged drinks and snacks that are low in calories but rich in vitamins and minerals. These pre-planned options make it easier to follow the diet without having to think too much about what to eat.

4. Stay Hydrated

Drinking plenty of water is a key part of the Hollywood Diet. Staying hydrated helps flush out toxins, keeps your energy up, and helps you feel full. The diet often recommends at least 8 glasses of water a day, sometimes along with herbal teas that act as natural diuretics to help reduce water weight.

5. Fruits and Veggies

A big part of the diet is eating lots of fruits and vegetables. These foods are low in calories but high in fiber, vitamins, and minerals. They help you stay full and get the nutrients you need without adding many calories.

6. Temporary Solution

Remember, the Hollywood Diet is a short-term fix, not a permanent lifestyle change. Its restrictive nature makes it hard to maintain for more than a few days. It's important to use it as a quick boost rather than a long-term plan.

7. Exercise Lightly

While the Hollywood Diet doesn't heavily focus on exercise, adding some light activities like walking, yoga, or stretching can help enhance your results. Light exercise can boost your metabolism and improve your overall sense of well-being without overwhelming your body during calorie restriction.

Making the Hollywood Diet Work for You

If you're thinking about trying the Hollywood Diet, here are a few tips to keep it safe and effective:

- Check with a Doctor: Before starting any new diet, especially one that's very restrictive, talk to a healthcare professional to make sure it's safe for you.

- Listen to Your Body: Pay attention to how you feel. If you start feeling dizzy, overly tired, or unwell, it's important to stop and consider a less restrictive approach.

- Use it as a Kick-Start: Think of the Hollywood Diet as a way to begin healthier eating habits. After you finish the diet, transition to a balanced, sustainable eating plan that includes a variety of foods from all food groups.

By understanding these principles and applying them thoughtfully, you can use the Hollywood Diet to achieve quick results while setting the foundation for a healthier lifestyle.

Here's the scoop on How It Really Works:

The Hollywood Diet has gained popularity thanks to its promise of quick weight loss, often endorsed by celebrities. Let's break down its key principles in a way that's relatable and easy to understand.

1. Calorie Restriction

The main idea behind the Hollywood Diet is to eat fewer calories than your body needs, creating a calorie deficit that leads to weight loss. Typically, this diet limits your intake to about 800-1200 calories a day. While this can help you lose weight fast, it's important to be careful and ensure you still get the nutrients your body needs.

2. Short-Term Focus

This diet isn't meant to be a long-term solution. It usually lasts from one day to a few days, providing a quick fix for those looking to shed pounds rapidly. Think of it as a way to jump-start your weight loss or to slim down quickly for a special event.

3. Pre-Planned Meals

The Hollywood Diet often includes specific meal plans or pre-packaged drinks and snacks that are low in calories but rich in vitamins and minerals. These pre-planned options make it easier to follow the diet without having to think too much about what to eat.

4. Stay Hydrated

Drinking plenty of water is a key part of the Hollywood Diet. Staying hydrated helps flush out toxins, keeps your energy up, and helps you feel full. The diet often recommends at least 8 glasses of water a day, sometimes along with herbal teas that act as natural diuretics to help reduce water weight.

5. Fruits and Veggies

A big part of the diet is eating lots of fruits and vegetables. These foods are low in calories but high in fiber, vitamins, and minerals. They help you stay full and get the nutrients you need without adding many calories.

6. Temporary Solution

Remember, the Hollywood Diet is a short-term fix, not a permanent lifestyle change. Its restrictive nature makes it hard to maintain for more than a few days. It's important to use it as a quick boost rather than a long-term plan.

7. Exercise Lightly

While the Hollywood Diet doesn't heavily focus on exercise, adding some light activities like walking, yoga, or stretching can help enhance your results. Light exercise can boost your metabolism and improve your overall sense of well-being without overwhelming your body during calorie restriction.

Making the Hollywood Diet Work for You

If you're thinking about trying the Hollywood Diet, here are a few tips to keep it safe and effective:

- Check with a Doctor: Before starting any new diet, especially one that's very restrictive, talk to a healthcare professional to make sure it's safe for you.

- Listen to Your Body: Pay attention to how you feel. If you start feeling dizzy, overly tired, or unwell, it's important to stop and consider a less restrictive approach.

- Use it as a Kick-Start: Think of the Hollywood Diet as a way to begin healthier eating habits. After you finish the diet, transition to a balanced, sustainable eating plan that includes a variety of foods from all food groups.

By understanding these principles and applying them thoughtfully, you can use the Hollywood Diet to achieve quick results while setting the foundation for a healthier lifestyle.

3

THE NUTRITIONAL PRINCIPLES OF

THE HOLLYWOOD DIET

The Hollywood Diet has gained a lot of attention with its promise of quick weight loss and glamorous results. To really understand it, let's look at its nutritional foundation and see how it works.

Basically, the Hollywood Diet is about drastically cutting down your calorie intake for a short period. It usually involves drinking specially formulated juices or shakes instead of eating regular meals.

These drinks are designed to give you the essential vitamins, minerals, and nutrients you need while keeping your calorie count very low. The idea is to create a calorie deficit so your body starts burning stored fat for energy.

While you might lose weight quickly on the Hollywood Diet, it's important to think about what this means for your nutrition. Since you're getting all your nutrients from these drinks, they need to be well-balanced. Ideally, they should provide enough protein, carbs, healthy fats, fiber, and a full range of vitamins and minerals. This way, even though you're cutting calories, your body still gets what it needs to function well.

However, not all meal replacement drinks are created equal. Some might not have all the nutrients you need, which could lead to deficiencies if you stick with the diet for too long. Plus, such a restrictive diet isn't usually sustainable. Rapid weight loss can often lead to quick weight gain once you go back to normal eating, especially if you haven't developed healthy eating habits.

The Hollywood Diet can be a useful tool if you need to lose a few pounds quickly for a special event. But for long-term results and overall health, it's better to adopt a balanced, sustainable approach to eating. This means incorporating whole foods, staying active, and developing healthy eating habits that you can maintain over time.

In conclusion, while the Hollywood Diet offers a way to lose weight quickly with a structured, nutrient-focused plan, it's important to be cautious and understand its limitations. Making sure any meal replacement products are nutrient-dense and using the diet as a starting point for healthier, more sustainable eating habits can help you achieve and maintain better health and your desired weight in the long run.

How the Hollywood Diet Impacts Your Metabolism

The Hollywood Diet, famous for its promise of rapid weight loss, has a significant impact on your metabolism. It's designed to produce quick results, often involving severe calorie restriction and specific meal replacements. While the allure of shedding pounds quickly can be tempting, it's important to understand how such a diet affects your body's metabolism.

When you drastically cut your calorie intake, your body goes into a sort of survival mode. Initially, you might see rapid weight loss, which can be motivating. However, this is often because your body is shedding water weight and burning through its glycogen stores. Once these are depleted, your metabolism starts to slow down to conserve energy, as it senses it's not getting enough fuel.

A slower metabolism means your body burns fewer calories at rest, making it harder to lose weight over time. This can lead to a plateau, where weight loss stalls despite continued efforts. Additionally, when you eventually return to a normal eating pattern, your slower metabolism can result in rapid weight gain, often leading to what's commonly known as "yo-yo dieting."

Moreover, the Hollywood Diet's restrictive nature can deprive your body of essential nutrients. This can lead to fatigue, muscle loss, and other health issues, as your body isn't receiving the balanced nutrition it needs to function optimally. Long-term reliance on such diets can also disrupt your relationship with food, making it harder to maintain a healthy lifestyle in the long run.

In essence, while the Hollywood Diet might offer quick weight loss, its impact on your metabolism can make sustainable weight management challenging. For lasting health benefits, a more balanced approach that includes a variety of foods, regular exercise, and mindful eating is far more effective. This way, you support your metabolism, nourish your body, and cultivate habits that promote long-term well-being.

Exploring the Good and Bad of the Hollywood Diet for Your Health

When it comes to trendy diets, the Hollywood Diet often grabs attention with its promise of fast weight loss. But like any diet, it has its own set of pros and cons that you should consider for your health.

Pros:

1. Quick Results: The biggest appeal of the Hollywood Diet is the promise of quick weight loss. If you have a special event coming up and want to lose a few pounds quickly, this diet can help you achieve that.

2. Simplicity: This diet is pretty straightforward. It often involves meal replacements like shakes or a specific meal plan, making it easier to follow without worrying about counting calories or figuring out complex meal plans.

3. Detox Effects: Many versions of the Hollywood Diet emphasize detoxing your body, which can help you cut out unhealthy foods and reduce bloating. Focusing on fresh fruits, vegetables, and staying hydrated can give your body a much-needed break from processed foods and excess salt.

Cons:

1. Short-Term Solution: The weight loss you achieve with the Hollywood Diet is often temporary. Once you go back to your regular eating habits, the weight is likely to come back, and sometimes you might gain even more.

2. Nutritional Gaps: Because the Hollywood Diet is so restrictive, you might miss out on important nutrients. Relying too much on meal replacements or a limited variety of foods can leave you lacking in essential vitamins and minerals.

3. Hunger and Fatigue: Rapid weight loss diets often make you feel hungry and tired. The Hollywood Diet is no different. With such a low-calorie intake, you might find yourself feeling exhausted and irritable, making it hard to stick to the diet for long.

4. Potential Health Risks: Extreme dieting can be tough on your body, leading to problems like

muscle loss, a weakened immune system, and even gallstones. It's important to approach any drastic diet change with caution and ideally under the guidance of a healthcare professional.

In the end, while the Hollywood Diet might seem like an appealing quick fix, it's crucial to weigh the potential health risks against the benefits. For long-term and healthy weight loss, a balanced diet combined with regular exercise is usually the best approach. Listen to your body and consider consulting with a nutritionist or doctor before starting any new diet plan.

4

PREPARING FOR THE HOLLYWOOD DIET

Starting the Hollywood Diet can feel both exciting and a bit overwhelming, but with the right approach, it can also be a rewarding journey toward better health.

First things first, let's understand what the Hollywood Diet is all about. It's designed to help you lose weight quickly by focusing on nutrient-rich foods and specific meal timings. You'll be eating lots of fruits, vegetables, lean proteins, and sometimes special diet products aimed at speeding up your weight loss.

To begin, set some clear and realistic goals for yourself. Think about why you want to try the Hollywood Diet and what you hope to achieve. Maybe you want to lose a certain amount of weight, fit into that favorite outfit, or simply feel more energetic. Having a clear goal will help keep you motivated.

Planning your meals and snacks is crucial. The Hollywood Diet requires mindful eating, so having a plan makes it easier to stick to. Stock up on fresh fruits and vegetables, lean meats, and any other foods the diet recommends. Prepping meals ahead of time can save you from last-minute temptations that might lead you off track.

It's wise to check in with a healthcare professional before starting any new diet, especially one that promises quick results. They can offer personalized advice and help you avoid any potential issues.

As you dive into the Hollywood Diet, remember to stay hydrated and pay attention to how your body feels. Rapid weight loss diets can be intense, so make sure you're getting enough nutrients and not pushing yourself too hard. Drink plenty of water, get enough rest, and take breaks if you need to.

Keeping a positive mindset is key. Changing your eating habits can be challenging, and it's normal to have ups and downs. Celebrate your progress, no matter how small, and don't beat yourself up if you have a slip-up. Every step forward is progress.

Getting Mentally Ready for the Hollywood Diet

Preparing yourself mentally for the Hollywood Diet is like gearing up for a big adventure. It's not just about what you eat; it's about getting your mind in the right place for the journey ahead.

First things first, set some realistic expectations. This diet isn't a magic fix; it's more of a kickstart to help you reach your goals. So, don't expect miracles overnight. Give yourself some grace and understand that it's a process.

Next, think about why you're doing this. Whether it's to feel healthier, look better, or just challenge yourself, reminding yourself of your "why" can keep you motivated when things get tough.

And speaking of tough, let's talk attitude. Having a positive mindset is key. Believe in yourself and your ability to stick to the plan. Surround yourself with people who support you and lift you up when you need it.

Now, let's be real—there will be bumps in the road. Temptations, cravings, maybe even a few slip-ups. But that's all part of it. The important thing is to stay focused on your goals and keep moving forward, no matter what.

So, as you get ready to dive into the Hollywood Diet, remember to get your head in the game. With the right mindset and a little determination, you've got this!

Setting Realistic Goals for the Hollywood Diet

When diving into the Hollywood Diet, setting goals that you can truly achieve is crucial. It's tempting to aim for the stars, envisioning a complete body transformation in record time. But hey, let's be real here.

Start by setting goals that are specific and within reach. Instead of fixating on dropping heaps of weight overnight, focus on smaller victories. Maybe it's shedding a few pounds or feeling more energized throughout the day. These are the goals that keep you motivated and moving forward.

And don't forget to stay flexible. The Hollywood Diet isn't a one-size-fits-all deal. If something's not working for you, it's okay to switch things up. Listen to your body and adjust your goals accordingly. It's all about finding what works best for you.

Oh, and celebrate those wins! Whether it's fitting into those jeans that were a bit snug last month or resisting that tempting slice of cake, give yourself a pat on the back. You deserve it!

But remember, the Hollywood Diet is just one piece of the puzzle. Pair it with regular exercise, good sleep, and managing stress, and you've got yourself a winning combo. It's all about finding balance and making sustainable changes for a healthier, happier you. You've got this!

5

THE HOLLYWOOD DIET MEAL PLAN

Let's chat about the Hollywood Diet plan! It's been making waves lately, especially with all those celebs endorsing it. Basically, it involves swapping out your regular meals for a special juice blend for a few days up to a week.

Now, some folks swear by it, but others approach it cautiously. I mean, who wouldn't be tempted by the idea of sipping on delicious juice instead of dealing with meal prep, right? But here's the thing: these liquid diets might leave you feeling pretty hungry and low on energy since they're often low in essential nutrients.

Sure, the Hollywood Diet can work wonders for some people, whether it's for a quick fix before a big event or as a kickstart to healthier habits. But it's not for everyone, and it's crucial to think about whether it fits into your lifestyle and health goals.

At the end of the day, rapid weight loss sounds appealing, but it's essential to think about the bigger picture. Your health and well-being should always come first, so take a moment to consider if the Hollywood Diet is the right choice for you. After all, we're all different, and what works for one person might not work for another!

Easy-to-Follow Calorie Guide for the Hollywood Diet

Let's talk about the nitty-gritty of calorie guidelines on the Hollywood Diet. Now, when you hear "Hollywood Diet," you might imagine strict calorie counting and deprivation, but it's not quite like that.

Here's the deal: while the Hollywood Diet does have its rules, it's not solely focused on slashing calories. Instead, it's more about what kinds of calories you're putting into your body. Think quality over quantity.

So, what are the guidelines? Well, it's all about balance and making smart choices. You want to load up on nutrient-dense foods like fruits, vegetables, lean proteins, and healthy fats. These foods not only keep you feeling satisfied but also provide your body with the fuel it needs to thrive.

Of course, portion control plays a role too. While you don't need to obsess over counting every single calorie, being mindful of your portions can help you stay on track and prevent overeating.

But here's the thing: the Hollywood Diet isn't about depriving yourself or feeling restricted. It's about finding a sustainable way of eating that works for you and makes you feel good inside and out.

So, go ahead, enjoy your meals, savor every bite, and trust that you're nourishing your body in the best possible way. That's what the Hollywood Diet is all about.

Workout Suggestionss for the Hollywood Diet

When you're diving into the Hollywood Diet, keeping up with workouts is a bit like adding the perfect seasoning to a dish – it's all about finding what works best for you. This diet focuses on shedding pounds fast with juice blends and calorie limits, so you want workouts that complement this without leaving you feeling drained.

1. Easy Does It with Cardio: Think low-impact cardio, like taking a brisk walk, a leisurely bike ride, or a refreshing swim. These keep the calorie burn going without putting too much strain on your body, which is crucial when your food choices are limited.

2. Muscle Matters: Don't forget to show your muscles some love with strength training. Bodyweight exercises are your friends here – squats, lunges, push-ups, and planks are all great. You can do them practically anywhere, even in your living room during commercial breaks.

3. Find Your Zen with Yoga and Pilates: Stretching it out with yoga or getting your core fired up with Pilates are awesome additions to your Hollywood Diet journey. They not only help with flexibility and strength but also do wonders for stress relief – something we all need when we're watching what we eat.

4. Spice Things Up with Intervals: If you're feeling up for a challenge, sprinkle some interval training into your routine. It's like a flavor explosion for your workout – short bursts of intense effort followed by rest or lower-intensity activity. It's efficient and helps boost your fitness level.

5. Listen to Your Body: Most importantly, tune in to what your body's telling you. If you're feeling wiped out, it's totally okay to dial back or take a day off. The Hollywood Diet can be pretty intense, so give yourself the downtime you need to stay strong and avoid burnout.

Just like crafting the perfect recipe, finding the right balance of diet and exercise takes some experimentation. Stick with what feels good and mix things up when you need a change. With a little creativity and consistency, you'll be rocking your Hollywood Diet journey feeling healthy, energized, and ready to tackle anything.

6
WHAT TO EAT AND AVOID

lright, let's chat about what's on the menu and what's off-limits when you're diving into the Hollywood Diet. Think of it as your backstage pass to the diet scene!

So, what's the star of the show? Fresh fruits and veggies steal the spotlight, giving you a burst of nutrients and keeping you feeling full and fabulous. And don't forget about the lean proteins like chicken, fish, and tofu—they're your trusty sidekicks, helping you stay strong and satisfied throughout the day.

Now, onto the villains—the foods you'll want to dodge. Sugary snacks and refined carbs are the bad guys here, messing with your energy levels and leaving you feeling like you've hit a red carpet slump. And processed foods? They're like the paparazzi of the diet world, full of sneaky additives and preservatives that you're better off without.

But hey, nobody's perfect, right? So if you find yourself reaching for that slice of pizza or indulging in a sweet treat, don't sweat it. The Hollywood Diet is all about finding your balance and feeling your best, so go ahead and enjoy the occasional splurge. After all, life's too short to skip the good stuff!

Sample Daily Menu

Breakfast:

Kickstart your day with a delicious fruit smoothie. Blend up your favorite fruits—think bananas, strawberries, and maybe even a handful of spinach—with some almond milk for a creamy, refreshing start to your morning.

Mid-Morning Snack:

When that mid-morning hunger hits, grab a handful of mixed nuts or slice up some crunchy veggies like carrots and bell peppers. Dip 'em in some hummus for an extra flavor kick that'll keep you going until lunchtime.

Lunch:

Time for a vibrant salad packed with all the good stuff! Load up your bowl with leafy greens, juicy cherry tomatoes, creamy avocado, and whatever other veggies you fancy. Add some grilled chicken or tofu on top for a protein boost, then drizzle with your favorite dressing.

Afternoon Pick-Me-Up:

Feeling a bit sluggish in the afternoon? Brew yourself a hot cup of green tea or crack open a cold coconut water. It'll perk you up and keep you hydrated without any added sugar or caffeine jitters.

Dinner:

For dinner, let's keep it hearty but healthy. How about some grilled salmon with a side of roasted sweet potatoes and steamed broccoli? It's a satisfying meal that's full of flavor and nutrients to fuel you through the evening.

Evening Treat:

Wrap up your day with a little something sweet. Treat yourself to a square of dark chocolate or a bowl of fresh fruit—it's the perfect way to satisfy your sweet tooth without going overboard.

Remember, the Hollywood Diet is all about nourishing your body with delicious, nutritious foods that leave you feeling great inside and out. So dig in and enjoy every bite!

Balancing Social Life and Diet

Finding the right balance between your social life and sticking to the Hollywood Diet can be a real challenge—it's like trying to juggle a bunch of oranges without dropping any. You want to enjoy hanging out with friends without feeling like you're missing out or sabotaging your health goals.

Picture this: you're at a friend's birthday bash, and there's a table full of tempting treats staring you down. It's like they're whispering, "Come on, just one won't hurt." We've all been there! But staying committed to your diet doesn't mean you have to miss out on the fun. It's about finding that sweet spot between indulging a little and staying on track.

One trick is to be strategic with your choices. Scope out the scene and look for healthier options, like veggie platters or grilled goodies. And if you can't resist that slice of cake or handful of chips, don't beat yourself up over it. Tomorrow's a new day, and you can get back on track with your diet then.

Communication is key, too. Let your friends know why you're eating the way you are and ask for their support. Chances are, they'll have your back and might even jump on board with you. After all, what's better than having a squad that's got your health in mind?

At the end of the day, it's all about finding that happy medium. You can enjoy hanging out with your pals and treat yourself now and then without derailing your progress. So go ahead, live it up—just remember to keep your eye on the prize and listen to what your body's telling you.

7

HOLLYWOOD DIET RECIPES FOR WEIGHT LOSS

DELIGHTFUL RECIPES FOR BREAKFAST

Pumpkin Pie Pancakes

INGREDIENTS

2 cups all-purpose flour

1 1/2 teaspoons baking powder

1/2 teaspoon baking soda

1/2 teaspoon kosher salt

3 tablespoons packed brown sugar

1 1/2 teaspoons ground cinnamon

1/4 teaspoon ground ginger

1/4 teaspoon freshly grated nutmeg

1 3/4 cups buttermilk

1 cup canned pumpkin purée (I prefer Libby)

2 large egg yolks

1 teaspoon vanilla extract

2 large egg whites

Canola oil (or another other neutral oil), for cooking

Powdered sugar, maple syrup, butter, and whipped cream, for serving

METHOD

Place the flour, baking powder, baking soda, salt, brown sugar, and spices in a medium bowl and whisk to combine.

Place the buttermilk, pumpkin purée, egg yolks, and vanilla in a blender and blend until smooth. Pour into the flour mixture and stir until almost combined, but with a few clumps of flour still remaining. Stir the reserved egg whites into the mixture until just combined. Set the batter aside to rest for about 10 minutes. Meanwhile, heat the skillet.

Heat about a tablespoon of oil in a large cast iron skillet or griddle on medium-high heat until shimmering. Add 1/4 cup portions of batter to the pan, pressing it out with the bottom of the measuring cup to help it spread out a bit. Reduce the heat to medium and cook until the bottoms are golden brown and a bit crispy, 1 to 2 minutes. Flip the pancakes and continue cooking until set, 2 to 2 1/2 minutes more. (I like to do a small test pancake to adjust the temperature before cooking the remaining batter.) Re-heat the griddle before cooking additional batches of pancakes.

Serve the pumpkin pie pancakes with a heavy dusting of powdered sugar, a drizzle of maple syrup, a slap of butter, and a pile of whipped cream.

Breakfast Sangria

INGREDIENTS

1 pink grapefruit

1 navel orange

2 limes

1 cup Cointreau

1 750ml bottle Prosecco

12 to 24 ounces plain or grapefruit sparkling water

METHOD

Slice the citrus fruit into half moons. Mix with the Cointreau in a pitcher that holds at least quarts. Add the Prosecco and cover the pitcher tightly with plastic wrap. Refrigerate overnight.

When ready to serve, top off the pitcher with sparkling water and serve with lime or orange wedges.

Roasted Garlic and Herb No-Knead Bread

Save to My Recipes

PRINT

 RECIPE

PREP TIME

15 minutes

COOK TIME

45 minutes

MAKES

1 loaf

SERVES

10 to 12

NUTRITIONAL INFO

VIEW

INGREDIENTS

3 cups all-purpose flour

1 teaspoon kosher salt

3/4 teaspoon active dry yeast

1 1/2 cups warm water

1 large head garlic

1 tablespoon fresh thyme leaves

2 teaspoons finely chopped fresh rosemary leaves

2 tablespoons olive oil

1 teaspoon flaky salt

METHOD

Measure 3 cups all-purpose flour, 1 teaspoon kosher salt, and 3/4 teaspoon active dry yeast into a large bowl and stir to combine. Make a well in the flour mixture, add 1 1/2 cups warm water to the well, and stir until a rough, shaggy dough forms. Cover the bowl and let the dough rise in a warm place until doubled in bulk and bubbly, 6 to 8 hours. Meanwhile, roast the garlic.

Arrange a rack in the middle of the oven and heat the oven to 400ºF. Remove the excess papery skins from 1 large head garlic and slice a thin layer off the top to expose the cloves. Wrap the garlic completely in aluminum foil and bake until tender, about 30 minutes. Let cool completely, then squeeze the roasted cloves out of their skins and reserve.

Lightly flour a piece of parchment paper and turn the dough out onto it. Sprinkle the dough with the roasted garlic cloves, 1 tablespoon fresh thyme leaves, and 2 teaspoons finely chopped fresh rosemary leaves. Fold the dough over onto itself 4 times to incorporate the add ins. Flip the dough over and quickly shape it into a tight, round ball.

Cover with a towel and let rise until nearly doubled in size, 1 to 1 1/2 hours. About 30 minutes before the dough is ready, arrange a rack in the middle of the oven, remove any racks above it, and heat the oven to 450°F. Place a large Dutch oven and its lid in the oven while it is heating.

Remove the Dutch oven from the oven. Using the parchment paper as a sling, carefully transfer the dough into the Dutch oven. Quickly drizzle the loaf with 2 tablespoons olive oil and sprinkle with 1 teaspoon flaky salt.

Cover the Dutch oven, place it back in the oven, and bake for 30 minutes. Uncover and bake until the top is browned, about 15 minutes more. Another way to know that the bread is ready is if an instant-read thermometer inserted into the top or side registers 210°F. Remove the Dutch oven from the oven and use the parchment paper to transfer the bread to a wire rack. Cool at least 15 minutes before slicing the bread.

Kale, Bacon & Egg Whole-Wheat Breakfast Sandwich

INGREDIENTS

1 whole-wheat bun

Mayonnaise or softened butter (optional)

1 strip bacon

1 1/2 cups kale, chopped into 1/2-inch ribbons

1 clove garlic, minced

1/4 teaspoon white wine vinegar

1 tablespoon vegetable oil

1 large egg

METHOD

Toast the bun and set it on a plate. Spread with mayonnaise or butter, if desired.

In a medium skillet, cook the bacon until crisp, and set aside on a paper towel-lined plate. Pour off the bacon grease, leaving just a thin film on the pan. Add the garlic and kale to the skillet and cook over medium-high heat, tossing frequently and scraping up any browned bits from the bottom of the pan. Taste and add salt if needed. Cook until kale is tender, adding 1 or 2 tablespoons of water if needed to keep kale moist as it cooks. Sprinkle with vinegar, then remove from pan and set aside.

Wipe skillet clean and add vegetable oil (or 1 tablespoon of reserved bacon grease, if you're feeling frisky). Over medium heat, fry the egg.

While it cooks, assemble the rest of the sandwich: Place the kale on the bottom half of the bun. Cut the bacon in half crosswise and place on top of the kale.

Top the kale and bacon with the fried egg and the top bun. Serve immediately, cutting in half just before eating.

Christmas Morning Banana Strata

INGREDIENTS

6 eggs

8 ounces mascarpone cheese

1 vanilla bean, scraped

1/2 tablespoon vanilla extract

3 tablespoons sugar

1 3/4 cups whole milk

3 bananas

16 ounces white bread, cut into 1-inch pieces (about 9 cups)

PAM Original Cooking Spray

Toasted walnuts, for serving (optional)

METHOD

In a large bowl, whisk together the eggs, mascarpone, vanilla bean, vanilla extract, and sugar until smooth. Whisk in the milk until incorporated.

Slice two of the bananas into the mixture, add the bread pieces, and stir to coat.

Spray a 2-quart baking dish with PAM Original Cooking Spray and pour the bread and egg mixture into the dish, using the back of a spoon to gently press into the dish. Cover with aluminum foil and refrigerate overnight.

The next morning, preheat the oven to 350°F. Uncover the strata and bake until the top just begins to brown and the liquid is thick but not yet firm, 30-40 minutes. Wait fifteen minutes before topping with the last banana, sliced, and serving warm with walnuts if desired.

Slow Cooker Creamy Pumpkin Spice Oatmeal

INGREDIENTS

Cooking spray, olive oil, or coconut oil

2 tablespoons unsalted butter, divided

1 1/2 cups steel-cut oats

1 (15-ounce) can pumpkin purée

1 teaspoon ground ginger

1/2 teaspoon ground nutmeg

1/4 teaspoon ground cloves

4 cups water

2 cups whole milk

1/4 cup maple syrup

1 (3-inch) cinnamon stick

1 teaspoon vanilla extract

1/4 teaspoon salt

For serving: heavy cream, ground cinnamon, and additional maple syrup (optional)

METHOD

Coat the bottom and sides of a 4- to 6-quart slow cooker with cooking spray, olive oil, or coconut oil.

Melt 1 tablespoon of the butter over medium-high heat in a large saucepan or Dutch oven. Add the oats and stir frequently until lightly toasted, about 3 minutes. Push the oats up to the side of the pan and melt the remaining tablespoon of butter in the center of the pan. Add the pumpkin purée to the center of the pan and cook without stirring for 1 minute. Add the ginger, nutmeg, and cloves into the purée and cook, stirring occasionally, until the purée darkens slightly and the raw smell disappears, 3 to 4 minutes more.

Transfer the mixture to the prepared slow cooker. Add the water, milk, maple syrup, cinnamon stick, vanilla, and salt and stir well to combine.

Cover the slow cooker and cook on the LOW setting for 8 hours. When finished, much of the pumpkin purée will have separated from the oats — don't panic! Stir well with a wooden spoon to recombine everything, and remove the cinnamon stick before serving. Spoon the oatmeal into bowls and finish with a splash of heavy cream, a dusting of ground cinnamon, and a drizzle of maple syrup, if desired.

Green Smoothie with Spinach, Pear, and Ginger

INGREDIENTS

1 1/2 cups water (can substitute coconut water or milk of choice)

2 cups spinach, washed and dried

1 ripe pear, seeded and chopped

1 tablespoon fresh lemon juice

1 teaspoon freshly grated ginger

1 tablespoon ground flaxseed

Honey to taste, optional

Mint to garnish, optional

METHOD

Place all **Ingredients**in a blender and blend until smooth.

Lefse Potato Pancakes, Van Gogh, and Grandparents

INGREDIENTS

3 medium potatoes, peeled and quartered

3 tablespoons milk

1/2 stick of butter

1 teaspoon sugar

1 teaspoon salt

1 cup flour

METHOD

Place the peeled and quartered potatoes in a pot of boiling water and cook until tender. Drain and mash well until smooth. Place mashed potatoes in freezer until cooled.

Melt the butter and add the milk, sugar, and salt. Mix well and add to the chilled potatoes. Stir well and add flour until a thick dough is formed similar to a pie crust. On a very well floured surface with a floured rolling pin, roll out egg sized portions of the dough into very thin pancakes.

Place a griddle or frying pan on high heat but do not add any butter or oil. Place the pancake on the dry pan and cook for about one minute until golden spots appear. Flip and cook the other side for an additional minute. Continue this process with the rest of the dough.

Serve with butter and a sprinkling of sugar (also nice with a bit of cinnamon). Roll into a log and eat immediately.

Banana-Date Smoothie

INGREDIENTS

2 medium ripe bananas

1/4 cup pitted dried dates, such as Medjool

2 cups almond milk

2 teaspoons chia seeds, soaked if time allows (see Recipe Note)

1/2 teaspoon ground cardamom

1/2 medium lime, juiced

4 ice cubes

Pinch ground cinnamon

Pinch salt

METHOD

Place all the **Ingredients**in a blender and blend on high speed until smooth, about 1 minute. Divide between 2 cups and serve with a sprinkle of cinnamon and salt. Best if served immediately. (Makes about 4 cups total.)

Chai Latte

INGREDIENTS

2 cinnamon sticks, broken into pieces

2 teaspoons whole black peppercorns

10 whole cloves

6 green cardamom pods, cracked

4 cups water

1 (2-inch) piece fresh ginger, thinly sliced

2 tablespoons loose-leaf black tea, or 6 black tea bags

1/2 cup sweetener, such as brown sugar, honey, or maple syrup (optional)

3 cups cold whole milk, coconut milk, or other non-dairy milk

METHOD

Toast the spices. Place 2 cinnamon sticks, 2 teaspoons whole black peppercorns, 10 whole cloves, and 10 cracked green cardamom pods in a small saucepan over medium heat and toast, shaking the pan occasionally, until fragrant, 3 to 4 minutes. Meanwhile, thinly slice 1 (2-inch) piece of fresh ginger.

Brew the tea. Add 4 cups water and thinly sliced fresh ginger and bring to a simmer. Simmer for 5 minutes.

Steep the tea. Remove from heat and add 2 tablespoons loose-leaf black tea, or 6 black tea bags. Cover and steep for 10 minutes.

Sweeten the tea. While the tea is still warm, add 1/2 cup sweetener of your choice and stir until combined or dissolved.

Strain the tea. Strain the tea through a fine-mesh strainer into a pitcher or teapot. Discard the spices and tea leaves. Store in the refrigerator for future use, or keep it warm while you froth the milk.

Froth the milk. For whole milk, froth 3 cups cold milk by shaking it in a jar or by whisking it vigorously over medium-high heat. For non-dairy milks, use an immersion blender to froth before heating.

Heat the milk. Heat the frothed milk in a small saucepan over low heat until warm.

Serve. Pour 3/4 cup of the warm tea base into each mug. Add 1/2 cup of warmed milk and stir to combine. Top with a heaping spoonful of milk froth.

Savory Radish and Goat Cheese Muffins

INGREDIENTS

7 tablespoons unsalted butter, melted and cooled, divided

2 cups all-purpose flour

2 teaspoons baking powder

1/2 teaspoon baking soda

2 teaspoons salt

1 teaspoon garlic powder

2 large eggs, beaten

1 1/4 cups buttermilk

2 tablespoons honey

1 medium bunch radishes (about 2 cups), stems removed and julienned, divided

4 ounces goat cheese, crumbled

Fresh ground black pepper

METHOD

Preheat the oven to 375°F. Grease or line a 12-cup muffin tin with baking papers.

In a large bowl, whisk together the flour, baking powder, baking soda, salt, and garlic powder. In a medium bowl, mix together the eggs, buttermilk, 5 tablespoons of cooled butter, and honey. Add the wet **Ingredients** to the dry **Things Needed**, stirring until just combined. Fold in all but 2 tablespoons or so of the radishes and the goat cheese.

Spoon the batter into the muffin cups, filling each about 3/4 full. Top each muffin with a few pieces of reserved radish, fresh-ground black pepper, and a spoonful of the remaining melted butter. Bake for 20 to 25 minutes, until tops just begin to brown, and a toothpick inserted in the center of a muffin comes out clean.

DELIGHTFUL RECIPES FOR LUNCH

Gingery Poached Egg Soup

INGREDIENTS

1 tablespoon toasted Asian sesame oil or vegetable oil

5 (1/4-inch) thick slices fresh ginger

2 cloves garlic, very thinly sliced

6 cups low-sodium chicken or vegetable broth

2 tablespoons tamari or soy sauce

12 ounces regular bok choy, Shanghai bok choy, or Napa cabbage

4 large eggs

Thinly sliced scallions, shichimi togarashi, or furikake, for garnish (optional)

METHOD

Heat the oil in a Dutch oven or wide pot over medium-high heat until shimmering. Add the ginger and garlic and cook, stirring constantly, until the garlic is just golden-brown around the edges, about 1 minute.

Carefully add the broth and tamari or soy sauce (it may sputter) and bring to a boil. Meanwhile, trim the stem ends from the bok choy or cabbage. If using Napa cabbage or large bok choy, cut into 1 1/2-inch pieces.

Add the bok choy or cabbage to the boiling soup, stir to combine, and bring back to a boil. Lower the heat to maintain a simmer and crack the eggs into the soup, keeping the eggs as far apart from each other as possible. Simmer undisturbed until the whites are set but the yolks are still runny, 3 to 4 minutes. Serve immediately, topped with scallions, shichimi togarashi, or furikake if desired.

Coconut Rice

INGREDIENTS

2 cups jasmine rice

2 1/2 cups boiling water

1 cup coconut milk, stirred

1 to 2 teaspoons sugar, or to taste

1 teaspoon salt, plus more to taste

3 makrut lime leaves, bruised

METHOD

Place the rice in a large bowl and rinse thoroughly, several times, until the water runs clear.

Place the boiling water, coconut milk, sugar, salt, and lime leaves in a heavy 2-quart pot, and warm over medium-high heat until the mixture starts to simmer. Add the rice and bring back to a low simmer. Cover the pot tightly with aluminum foil or a tight-fitting lid, then turn the heat down to low.

Cook, undisturbed, for about 15 minutes, then turn off the heat and let the rice steam for another 5 to 10 minutes. Uncover, fluff, and serve.

Southwestern-Spiced Pork Tenderloin

INGREDIENTS

2 to 2 1/2 pounds pork tenderloin (usually 2 tenderloins)

1 tablespoon chili powder

1 tablespoon cumin

1 tablespoon smoked paprika

2 teaspoons cinnamon

2 teaspoons kosher salt

1 1/2 teaspoons freshly ground black pepper

1 teaspoon vegetable oil

METHOD

Preheat the oven to 450°F. Place a cast iron skillet
or roasting pan in the oven as it is heating.

Pat the pork dry and cut off any large pieces of surface fat. Mix together all the spices in a small bowl and rub them into the surface of the pork on all sides.

Remove the hot pan from the oven and swirl the oil to coat the bottom. Set the pork in the pan and return the pan to the oven. Roast for 10 minutes, and then flip the pork to the other side. Reduce the oven temperature to 400°F and continue roasting another 10 to 15 minutes, until the internal temperature of the pork registers 140°F to 145°F in the thickest part of the meat (20 to 25 minutes total).

Transfer the pork to a cutting board, tent with foil, and let it rest for 10 minutes before slicing. For extra-thin slices for sandwiches, cool the pork completely, then refrigerate before cutting.

Leftovers will keep for one week refrigerated.

Couscous Salad with Cucumber, Red Onion &
Herbs

THINGS NEEDED

1 cup couscous

1 1/4 cups boiling water

1 cup loosely packed cilantro, finely chopped

1 cup loosely packed Italian parsley, finely chopped

1/2 English cucumber, cut lengthwise and very
thinly sliced

1/2 red onion, cut in half and shaved extremely thin

1 lemon, zested and juiced, about 3 tablespoons

1/4 cup extra-virgin olive oil

1 tablespoon honey or agave syrup, warmed

1/2 teaspoon chili powder

1/2 teaspoon ground cumin

3 tablespoons toasted pine nuts

3 ounces feta cheese, optional

Salt and pepper, to taste

METHOD

Put the couscous in a large bowl and pour the boiling water over it. Cover with a lid or a plate and set aside for 5 minutes. Then remove the lid and fluff with a fork.

Toss the finely chopped herbs with the couscous, as well as the sliced cucumber, onion, and lemon zest.

Whisk together the lemon juice, olive oil, honey, chili powder, and cumin, then toss this dressing with the couscous. Stir in the pine nuts. Crumble the feta and stir that in as well. Taste and season generously with salt and pepper.

Serve immediately, or refrigerate until ready to serve. Store leftovers in a covered container for up to 5 days.

Hearts of Palm, Corn, Tomatoes & Watercress Salad

INGREDIENTS

1 head butter lettuce, washed and torn into large pieces

1 bunch watercress, washed and trimmed

1 1/2 cups sliced hearts of palm

1 1/2 cups fresh corn

2 cups cherry tomatoes

1 shallot, sliced thin

2 cups roasted potatoes (I used a Russet but small, red potatoes would be more like what they served in Chile)

1 cup green olives

olive oil and lemon to taste

salt and pepper to taste

METHOD

To assemble the salad, prep all the **Ingredients**and plate keeping everything separate.

Dress with olive oil, lemon, salt and pepper to taste. Serve immediately.

Potato Salad with Yogurt, Arugula, and Dill

INGREDIENTS

1 1/2 pounds new potatoes, cleaned

Salt

Freshly ground black pepper

1/2 cup whole milk plain yogurt

1/4 cup mayonnaise

2 large shallots, peeled and thinly sliced

1 large bunch arugula leaves, coarsely chopped

1 small bunch fresh dill, finely chopped

METHOD

Fill a 4-quart or larger pot halfway with water. Salt generously with at least 1 tablespoon of salt. Bring to a boil over high heat and add the potatoes. Bring back to a simmer and then turn the heat down to medium. Cook until the potatoes can be easily pierced with a fork, 15 to 20 minutes. Drain the potatoes and return them to the pot.

Use a fork to pull a hot potato out of the pot, and slice it into quarters. Repeat with the rest of the potatoes, adding them to a large bowl as you cut them up.

Whisk together the yogurt and mayonnaise. Toss the potatoes with this dressing, then toss with the shallots, arugula, and dill. Season to taste with salt and pepper. Refrigerate for at least 1 hour before serving.

Instant Pot Chicken Noodle Soup

INGREDIENTS

1 large yellow onion

3 stalks celery

3 medium carrots

2 cloves garlic

2 tablespoons olive oil

1 1/2 teaspoons kosher salt

1/4 teaspoon freshly ground black pepper

1 teaspoon dried thyme

2 bay leaves

1 1/2 pounds boneless, skinless chicken thighs

1 (32-ounce) box low-sodium chicken broth (4 cups)

2 cups water

1/4 cup fresh parsley leaves

2 tablespoons freshly squeezed lemon juice (from 1/2 medium lemon)

6 ounces extra-wide dried egg noodles (about 4 heaping cups)

METHOD

Prepare the following vegetables, adding them all to the same bowl: Dice 1 large yellow onion (about 2 cups) and 3 medium celery stalks (about 1 cup); peel and cut 2 medium carrots into 1/2-inch thick rounds (about 1 1/2 cups). Mince 2 garlic cloves and set aside separately.

Heat 2 tablespoons olive oil in a 6-quart or larger electric pressure cooker or Instant Pot with the Sauté function. Tlt the insert to coat with the oil. Add the onion, celery, carrot, 1 1/2 teaspoons kosher salt, and 1/4 teaspoon black pepper. Cook, stirring occasionally, until the vegetables are tender, 6 to 8 minutes. Stir in the garlic, 1 teaspoon dried thyme, and 2 bay leaves, and cook for 1 minute more. Turn the pressure cooker off. Add 1 1/2 pounds boneless, skinless chicken thighs, 1 box chicken broth, and 2 cups water.

Lock on the lid and make sure the pressure valve is set to seal. Set to cook for 10 minutes under HIGH pressure. It will take about 20 minutes to come up to pressure. Meanwhile, coarsely chop 1/4 cup parsley leaves and squeeze 2 tablespoons lemon juice.

When the cook time is up, let the pressure naturally release for 10 minutes. Quick release any remaining pressure. Transfer the chicken with tongs to a clean cutting board. Remove and discard the bay leaves.

Turn the pressure cooker back on to Sauté and bring the soup to a boil. Add 6 ounces egg noodles (about 4 heaping cups) and cook uncovered until just tender, about 5 minutes. Meanwhile, shred the chicken with two forks.

Return the shredded chicken to the pot and stir in the parsley and lemon juice. Serve immediately.

Tomato Tarte Tatin

INGREDIENTS

1 tablespoon olive oil

2 pints cherry tomatoes (about 4 cups), preferably a mix of colors

Kosher salt

Freshly ground black pepper

2 tablespoons balsamic vinegar

1 teaspoon honey

2 teaspoons chopped fresh thyme leaves, plus a handful of small sprigs for garnish

1 sheet frozen puff pastry (7 to 9 ounces, from one 1-pound box that contains 2 sheets), thawed but still cold, and corners cut off to make very rough 9- to 10-inch round

METHOD

Arrange a rack in the middle of the oven and heat to 400°F.

Heat the oil in an ovenproof 9- or 10-inch skillet, preferably cast iron, over medium heat until shimmering. Add the tomatoes and season lightly with salt and pepper. Cook, stirring once or twice, and as tomatoes begin to pop and release their juices, use a slotted spoon to press each down gently to release even more of their juice, then transfer them to a plate. All of the tomatoes should have popped after 8 to 10 minutes. Remove the pan from the heat (do not clean) and let the tomatoes cool on the the plate to the touch, 5 to 10 minutes.

Once the tomatoes are cool enough to handle, return the skillet to medium heat and add the vinegar and honey. Bring the mixture to a simmer and cook until reduced slightly, thick, and syrupy, about 1 minute.

Remove the skillet from the heat. Use your fingers to gently return the tomatoes to the skillet in one even layer, nestling them beside each other to fit as needed. Leave any juices that have collected on the plate behind. Sprinkle the chopped thyme over the tomatoes along with another big pinch of salt and a few grinds of black pepper.

Place the puff pastry round on top of the tomatoes, folding under any edges, if needed. Prick the pastry with a fork in a handful of spots.

Bake until the puff pastry is golden-brown, 25 to 30 minutes. Remove from the oven, let stand for 5 minutes, then run a knife around the pastry to loosen it from the pan. Invert a large plate over the top of the skillet and, using oven mitts, carefully and quickly flip the tarte tatin onto the plate. Rearrange any tomatoes that may have fallen out of place. Garnish with the thyme sprigs and serve warm or at room temperature, cut into wedges.

French Onion Frittata

INGREDIENTS

2 tablespoons unsalted butter, divided

2 cups diced day-old bread

1 tablespoon olive oil

2 large yellow onions, thinly sliced

1 1/2 teaspoons kosher salt, divided

1 tablespoon balsamic vinegar

8 large eggs

1/4 cup whole or 2% milk

1 tablespoon Dijon mustard

1/4 teaspoon freshly ground black pepper

1/2 cup diced Gruyère cheese (2 ounces)

1 tablespoon finely chopped fresh chives

METHOD

Arrange a rack in the middle of the oven and heat to 400°F.

Heat 1 tablespoon of the butter in a 10-inch cast iron skillet over medium heat until bubbling. Add the bread cubes to the pan, toss to coat with the butter, and arrange in a single layer. Toast the bread, tossing every minute or so, until the bread cubes are golden-brown on all sides, about 5 minutes total. Transfer the croutons to a bowl; set aside.

Reduce the heat to low. Add the oil, onions, and 1/2 teaspoon of the salt to the same skillet. Cook, stirring every 5 to 10 minutes and scraping any browned build-up from the bottom of the pan, until the onions are soft and deeply browned, about 40 minutes total. Add the vinegar and scrape up the browned bits at the bottom of the pan.

Whisk together the eggs, milk, mustard, remaining 1 teaspoon salt, and pepper in a large bowl. Stir the remaining butter and croutons into the skillet, then spread in an even layer. Pour the egg mixture over the top. Tilt the pan to make sure the eggs settle evenly. Top with the cheese. Cook until the eggs at the edges of the skillet begin to set, 2 to 4 minutes.

Bake until the eggs are set, 8 to 10 minutes. To check, cut a small slit in the center of the frittata. If raw eggs run into the cut, bake for another few minutes; if the eggs are set, pull the frittata from the oven.

Cool in the pan for 5 minutes, top with chives, then slice into wedges and serve warm.

Chilled Cucumber Noodles with Sesame Dressing

INGREDIENTS

2 large cucumbers (about 1 pound), peeled

1/2 teaspoon kosher salt, plus more as needed

2 tablespoons rice vinegar

1 tablespoon Asian sesame oil

1 teaspoon granulated sugar (optional)

Toasted sesame seeds (optional)

METHOD

Fit a colander or fine-mesh strainer over a large bowl. Using a spiralizer with the thinnest "noodle" attachment, spiralize the cucumber into long, thin strands. Place in the colander, sprinkle with the 1/2 teaspoon salt, and toss to combine. Let the noodles stand 30 minutes at room temperature.

Meanwhile, whisk together the vinegar, sesame oil, and sugar in a large mixing bowl until the sugar is dissolved.

When the noodles are ready, add them to the dressing and gently toss to coat. Taste and season with more salt as needed. Sprinkle with toasted sesame seeds if using and serve immediately.

Wild Rice Burgers

INGREDIENTS

1/2 cup uncooked wild rice (or 1 1/3 cups cooked wild rice)

2 tablespoons olive oil, divided

1/3 cup small-diced onion

1/3 cup small-diced celery

1 clove garlic, minced

1/2 cup fresh or panko breadcrumbs

1/4 cup shredded aged Asiago or Parmesan cheese

1/2 teaspoon kosher salt

1/2 teaspoon dried oregano

1/2 teaspoon dried thyme

1/4 teaspoon paprika

1/8 teaspoon cayenne pepper

1/16 teaspoon black pepper

2 large eggs, beaten

Burger buns and toppings (optional)

METHOD

If you are using uncooked wild rice, cook it according to package **Method** or use the boiling **Method**. Cool completely. (Can make a day ahead and refrigerate.)

Heat 1 tablespoon olive oil in a nonstick skillet over medium-low heat and sauté onions, celery, and garlic until onion is translucent. Set the skillet aside (no need to wash).

In a large bowl, combine onion-celery-garlic mixture with wild rice, breadcrumbs, cheese, salt, oregano, thyme, paprika, cayenne, and black pepper. Cool completely and then add eggs, stirring to combine.

Divide the mixture into 4 portions and shape each into 1/2-inch-thick patties.

Heat the remaining tablespoon of olive oil in the nonstick skillet over medium heat. Fry patties 2 to 3 minutes on each side until crisp and golden.

Serve with your favorite burger toppings.

Asian Cauliflower Fried Rice with Kalua Pork

INGREDIENTS

1 small head cauliflower, separated in florets

2 large eggs

1 (1-inch) piece ginger, peeled and grated with a microplane

1 small yellow onion, minced

4 ounces sliced mushrooms

1/4 to 1/2 cup Kalua pork (or substitute 3 strips bacon, fried and crumbled, or any other leftover meat)

2 scallions, thinly sliced

2 tablespoons chopped cilantro leaves

2 tablespoons chopped basil

1 tablespoon chopped mint

1 to 2 tablespoons coconut aminos

Kosher salt

Freshly ground black pepper

Splash of coconut vinegar (optional)

Splash of fish sauce (not optional)

METHOD

First, pulse the cauliflower in a food processor until
the pieces are the size of rice and chop the rest of
the **Things Needed**. Whisk the two eggs in a small
bowl with some salt and pepper to taste.

Warm a little bacon grease or other cooking fat in a
large cast iron skillet over medium heat. Pour the
whisked eggs into the hot pan and fry a thin egg
omelet. Take the egg out of the pan, slice it thinly,
and set it aside.

I always keep a large knob of ginger on hand in my freezer. It keeps really well. When I need to use it, I take it out of the freezer, peel off the skin with my vegetable peeler, and microplane it. It's almost like making ginger-flavored shaved ice.

Crank up the heat under your cast iron skillet to medium-high and add the chopped onions (along with a dash of salt and pepper). Once the onion softens, toss in the sliced mushrooms and Kalua pork (along with yet another sprinkle of salt and pepper), and stir-fry everything until the mushrooms are browned.

Add the ginger and stir it around for 30 seconds, then throw in the cauliflower and even more salt and pepper. Put a lid on the skillet and lower the heat to low and cook covered for about 5 minutes. When the cauliflower is tender (but not too mushy), add the coconut aminos, herbs, and sliced egg omelet. You can also add a little coconut vinegar to add a tiny bit of tang to the dish. And splash on some fish sauce for good measure.

Voila!

Tortellini Salad with Figs, Walnuts, Prosciutto & Greens

INGREDIENTS

1 (10-ounce) container fresh cheese tortellini

1/2 cup walnuts

1/2 cup dried Mission figs, stems removed (swap in fresh figs if you have them!)

4 slices prosciutto

5 ounces salad greens (about 5 big handfuls)

2 to 4 tablespoons balsamic vinaigrette

METHOD

Bring a pot of water to a boil over high heat. Add a teaspoon of salt and the tortellini, and cook until the tortellini bob to the surface and are tender, 6 to 8 minutes. Drain and set aside.

Meanwhile, heat the oven to 350°F. Spread the walnuts on a baking sheet and toast until fragrant and beginning to brown, 5 to 7 minutes. Transfer to a cutting board and roughly chop once cool enough to handle.

Trim the stems from the Mission figs and roughly chop. Tear the pieces of prosciutto into long ribbons.

Combine the cooked tortellini, figs, prosciutto, and salad greens in a bowl. Toss with enough balsamic vinaigrette to coat — start with 2 tablespoons and add more to taste. Divide the salad between serving bowls and sprinkle the walnuts on top.

DELIGHTFUL RECIPES FOR DINNER

Sauerkraut, Potato & Cheese Pierogi

INGREDIENTS

PIEROGI DOUGH:

3 cups all-purpose flour, plus extra as needed

1 teaspoon salt

1 large egg

1/4 cup sour cream

3/4 cup water

PIEROGI FILLING:

1 pound potatoes (I prefer red-skinned, but russet or yukon golds are fine)

2 tablespoons sour cream

1/4 teaspoon salt

1 cup drained sauerkraut

2 cups shredded sharp cheddar cheese

TO SERVE:

3 tablespoons butter

1 small yellow onion, sliced thinly

METHOD

To make the dough, whisk together the flour and salt in the bowl of a standing mixer (or regular mixing bowl). Whisk together the egg, sour cream, and water until combined, and then pour over the flour. Stir together the liquids and the flour with a wooden spoon or spatula until a shaggy dough is formed.

Knead the dough the mixer on low speed with the dough hook attachment until the dough is very smooth and soft, about 5 minutes. Alternatively, knead by hand against the counter for 8 minutes. If the dough seems very sticky after a few minutes of kneading, add a tablespoon of flour at a time until it starts coming together into a smooth ball. Cover and set aside to rest on the counter while you make the filling.

To make the filling, scrub the potatoes clean and place them in a 2- or 4-quart sauce pan. Cover with an inch or two of water and set over high heat. When the water comes to a boil, reduce the heat to medium-low and simmer until the potatoes are tender when pierced by a fork, 6 to 10 minutes depending on the size of your potatoes.

Transfer the potatoes to a mixing bowl with a slotted spoon. Remove the peels if desired (I like to leave them on!). Mash the potatoes into large chunks with a potato masher or a dinner fork. Add the sour cream and salt, and continue mashing until the potatoes are smooth. Add the sauerkraut and cheese, and stir to combine. Taste and add more salt if needed.

Shape the filling into 1" balls (roughly the diameter of a quarter) and arrange them on a dinner plate.

Pre-shaping the filling makes it easier and quicker to shape the pierogi.

Line a baking sheet with parchment and sprinkle generously with flour. Set this near your workspace.

Divide the pierogi dough in half, working with one half at a time and keeping the other half covered. Sprinkle your work surface with flour and roll out the pierogi dough to 1/8" thick. Stop occasionally to lift the dough and make sure it's not sticking to the work surface; use more flour as needed. If the dough shrinks back as you roll, let it sit for 5 minutes and then roll again.

Use a 3" biscuit cutter or drinking glass to cut the dough into rounds. Gather the scraps and set them aside.

To shape the pierogi, hold one of the rounds of dough in the palm of your hand and set a ball of filling in the middle. Fold the round in half, pinching it closed at the top and then working your way along the sides to form a half-moon shape. Make sure the edges of the dough are completely sealed. Set the pierogi on the floured baking sheet.

Continue to shape pierogi with the remaining rounds of dough. Lay them close together on the baking sheet, but don't let them touch. Roll out the second half of the dough, and cut and shape the pierogi as described. When finished, roll the scrapes and continue to make as many pierogi as you can. You should end up with roughly 4 dozen pierogi.→ Recipe Tip! No matter what, I always seem to end up with either a few leftover balls of filling or an extra bit of dough. C'est la vie! The balls are delicious eaten as a snack, even cold from the fridge. The scraps of dough can be rolled out, sliced into spaghetti-thin strips, and then boiled just like pasta for an afternoon snack.

At this point, the pierogi can be boiled and served right away or frozen. To freeze, place the sheet pan of pierogi in the freezer and freeze until solid. Transfer the frozen pierogi to a freezer container and freeze for up to three months. Pierogi can be cooked straight from the freezer.

When ready to cook the pierogi, melt the butter in a large skillet over medium heat. Add the onions and cook until the onions are translucent, very soft, and beginning to brown, 8 to 10 minutes. Push the onions to the edges of the pan where they will stay warm and continue to caramelize.

Meanwhile, bring a large pot of water to a boil. Salt generously. Working in batches, add 10 or so pierogi to the boiling water and stir to make sure they don't stick to the bottom. Cook the pierogi until all the pierogi have floated to the surface and then 1 to 2 minutes longer to make sure the filling gets hot — 8 to 10 minutes total.

Transfer the pierogi to the pan with the onions. Turn the heat to medium-high. Cook the pierogi without moving until they are golden and crispy on the bottoms, 2 to 3 minutes. If you're cooking more batches, transfer the pierogi to a serving dish. Once all the pierogi have been boiled and crisped, scrape the onions over the pierogi and gently stir to coat the pierogi with butter and onions. Serve immediately while hot.

Baked Beans with Pineapple and Bacon

INGREDIENTS

1 pound (about 2 1/4 cups) dried navy beans or Great Northern Beans

1/4 cup dark brown sugar

1/4 cup molasses

2 1/2 teaspoons dry mustard

1 teaspoon salt

1 (15-ounce can) diced tomatoes

1 cup crushed pineapple (canned in juice or fresh)

1 bunch green onions, sliced into 1/2-inch pieces

8 thick slices smoked bacon

METHOD

Rinse the beans and soak them in 6 cups of water overnight or at least 6 hours.*

Preheat the oven to 325°F.

Add beans with their soaking liquid to the pot. Combine the brown sugar, molasses, mustard, and salt, and pour the mixture over the beans. Add the tomatoes, pineapple, and all but 1/2 cup of the green onions. Stir the pot to combine the **Things Needed**. Lay the bacon strips across the top of the beans.

Cover the pot and bake about 5 hours, until the beans are tender but not falling apart and mushy.

Uncover during the last 30 minutes of cooking to allow the bacon to crisp.

Serve in bowls topped with a few pinches of sliced green onion.

One-Pot Braised Cabbage with Bacon

INGREDIENTS

5 thick-cut slices bacon, cut crosswise into 1/3-inch-thick pieces

Olive oil, if needed

5 cloves garlic, finely chopped

1 medium green cabbage (about 2 pounds), cut through the core into 1/4-inch-thick wedges

1 cup low-sodium chicken broth

1 bay leaf

1 1/2 teaspoons kosher salt

1 1/2 tablespoons apple cider vinegar

Kosher salt

Freshly ground black pepper

METHOD

Heat a 5-quart or larger Dutch oven on medium-high heat. Add the bacon and cook, stirring occasionally, until crispy and most of the fat is rendered, 8 to 10 minutes. Remove with a slotted spoon to a paper towel-lined plate. Take the pot off the heat and let cool a few minutes. If you have less than 3 tablespoons of grease in the pot, add olive oil to make up the difference.

Place the Dutch oven back over medium-high heat; add the garlic and stir. Place the cabbage wedges cut-side down in the pot (they will not sit in one layer). Cook undisturbed until the cabbage pieces on the bottom begin to slightly brown, 4 to 5 minutes. Using a wooden spoon, bring up the cabbage sitting on the bottom to rotate the pieces on the top to the bottom of the pot. Continue cooking until the cabbage slightly wilts and more pieces brown on the edges, 7 to 8 minutes.

Reduce the heat to medium. Add the broth, bay leaf, and salt. Simmer, stirring every few minutes, until the cabbage is tender and all the liquid is evaporated, 20 to 25 minutes.

Remove from the heat and stir in the vinegar. Taste and season with salt and pepper as needed. Scatter the crispy bacon on top and serve immediately.

Kale & Potato Soup

INGREDIENTS

1 medium (8 ounce) yellow or russet potato, scrubbed clean and chopped

1 clove garlic, minced

1/2 teaspoon kosher salt

2 cups vegetable stock, chicken stock, or water

1/2 bunch kale (6 to 8 big leaves), preferably dino, lacinato, or Tuscan

1 teaspoon lemon juice or cider vinegar

1 to 2 large eggs, depending on your appetite

Salt and pepper

Grated Parmesan cheese, extra-virgin olive oil, or yogurt, to serve

METHOD

Combine the chopped potato, garlic, salt, and stock (or water) in a medium saucepan over medium-high heat. Bring to a boil, then reduce the heat to simmer.

While the potatoes start to cook, chop the kale. Remove any thick, tough stems and chop them into small pieces. Add the chopped stems to the pot with the potatoes and simmer for 2 minutes.

Stack the leaves of kale on top of each other. Slice them crosswise into thin ribbons, and add them to the pot with the potatoes and kale stems. If necessary, add more stock or water to the pot to just about cover the kale.

Cover the pot and let the soup cook for 8 to 10 minutes. The soup is ready when the potatoes are easily pierced with a fork, and when a ribbon of kale has become tender, but has not yet become stringy or pulpy. Stir in the lemon juice or vinegar. Taste and season with more salt and fresh cracked pepper. Also add more stock or water if a more brothy soup is desired.

To finish, crack the eggs into measuring cups, and then gently slide them into the soup. Ladle some of the soup broth on top of the eggs to submerge them. Put the lid back on the pot and cook for 4 minutes. When done, the whites of the eggs should be opaque, but the yolk should still be soft. If the eggs break into the soup before they are poached, just use a fork to swirl them into the soup, like egg drop soup.

Carefully spoon the eggs into a soup bowl. Ladle the soup on top. Finish with a sprinkle of Parmesan cheese, a drizzle of olive oil, or a spoonful of yogurt.

Pasta with Cauliflower, Sausage & Breadcrumbs

INGREDIENTS

1/2 tablespoon olive oil

1 large shallot or small onion, diced

2 cloves garlic, minced

1/2 pound sweet Italian sausage

1 head cauliflower, cut into small, bite-sized florets

1 teaspoon salt

Pepper

2 (14.5-ounce) cans diced tomatoes

1 pound pasta, any shape

1/2 to 3/4 cup fresh breadcrumbs or panko

1/2 pound mozzarella, cut or shredded into small pieces

METHOD

Start a large pot of water to boiling over high heat for the pasta. It will take several minutes to come to a boil.

Meanwhile, heat the olive oil in a large, high-sided skillet over medium heat (use a 14-inch skillet if you have one). Add the shallot or onion, season with salt and pepper, and sauté until soft and translucent, 5 to 8 minutes. Add the garlic and cook until fragrant, about 30 seconds. Add the sausage, breaking it up as it cooks.

When the sausage is almost cooked through, add the cauliflower, salt, and pepper. Push the cauliflower down into the pan so the florets have as much surface contact with the pan as possible. Cook, stirring occasionally, until the cauliflower begins to brown slightly. If the pan is very dry, depending on how much fat is in your sausage, you can add another splash of oil.

Turn the heat up to medium-high and pour in the tomatoes. Scrape any brown bits off of the bottom of the pan. Bring the mixture to a simmer, then cover, lower the heat to medium-low, and simmer until the cauliflower is cooked through, about 10 minutes.

While the sauce is simmering, boil the pasta. When the pasta is al dente, drain it and set aside. Also, spread the breadcrumbs onto a cookie sheet and run under the broiler to lightly toast; alternatively, brown the breadcrumbs in a dry skillet.

If your pan is big enough, transfer the pasta to the pan with the sauce once the cauliflower is tender. Otherwise, combine everything in a large serving bowl. Toss together, then add the cubes of mozzarella.

Top each serving with breadcrumbs, reserving extra breadcrumbs for leftovers.

Braised Beef in Tomatoes & Red Wine

INGREDIENTS

5 pounds chuck roast

1 tablespoon peanut or vegetable oil

Salt and freshly ground black pepper

2 large yellow onions, diced

10 cloves garlic, minced

1/4 to 1/2 teaspoon red pepper flakes, optional

1 (32-ounce) can diced tomatoes, drained

2 cups bold red wine, such as Chianti

1/4 cup balsamic vinegar

METHOD

Heat the oven to 325°F. Cut the chuck roast into 3 or 4 large pieces. Brush the pieces with oil and apply salt and pepper generously. Heat your largest, deepest sauté pan over medium-high heat and sear the meat for several minutes on each side, about 12 minutes in all. (If the meat does not all fit in the sauté pan at once, do this in batches.) When the meat is well seared, with a dark brown crust all over, remove to a plate and turn the heat down to low.

Add the onions and garlic, and sprinkle with salt. Cook on low heat for 10 minutes or until they are golden and soft. Add the red pepper flakes, if you desire a little kick.

Stir in the diced tomatoes and sauté over medium heat for 2 to 3 minutes, then stir in the red wine. Bring to a simmer, scraping any browned bits off the bottom of the pan, then turn off the heat and stir in the balsamic vinegar. Put the chuck roast pieces back in the sauté pan. (If the pan is too small, transfer meat and sauce to a Dutch oven.)

Cover the pan and cook in the oven for 4 hours. (This can also be done in a slow cooker. At this point transfer to a slow cooker and cook on LOW 8 to 10 hours.)

After 4 hours, remove the meat from the oven and cool for 20 to 30 minutes. Use two forks to shred the meat thoroughly. Refrigerate overnight. The next day, scrape off the layer of fat that has hardened on top of the meat. The meat can be refrigerated for up to 3 days, and warmed gently in the oven for about an hour at 300°F.

The meat can be served as it is, in its sauciness, or you can pour off much of the sauce, and blend it into a smooth, thicker sauce. Serve over polenta or pasta with a good red wine

Oven-Roasted Frozen Broccoli

INGREDIENTS

1 (16-ounce) bag frozen broccoli florets (do not thaw)

2 tablespoons olive oil

1/2 teaspoon kosher salt

Freshly ground black pepper

1/4 cup grated Parmesan cheese

1 medium lemon, halved

METHOD

Arrange one rack in the middle of the oven and one rack in the highest position, then heat to 450°F. Place a rimmed baking sheet in the oven while it's heating.

Combine the broccoli, olive oil, salt, and a few grinds of pepper in a large bowl and toss to coat. Carefully remove the hot baking sheet from the oven, add the broccoli, and spread it into an even layer. Roast on the middle rack until the broccoli is tender and beginning to brown at the edges, 15 to 18 minutes.

Remove from the oven. Switch the oven to broil. Scatter the Parmesan evenly over the broccoli.

Return to the oven and broil on the upper rack until the cheese melts, 1 to 2 minutes. Squeeze the juice from one lemon half over the broccoli and toss to combine. Cut the other lemon half into wedges and serve alongside the broccoli.

Grilled veggie low carb plate

Things Needed

8 oz. eggplant

8 oz. zucchini

¼ cup olive oil

1 tbsp lemon juice

5 oz. (1¼ cups) cheddar cheese, cubed

10 black olives

1 oz. (3 tbsp) almonds

½ cup (3 oz.) Greek yogurt (4% fat)

1 cup (2 oz.) leafy greens

salt and pepper

Method

Slice eggplant and zucchini into half-inch-thick (1 cm) slices lengthwise. Salt on both sides and let them sit for 5-10 minutes.

Preheat the oven to 450°F (225°C), or, even better, set the oven to broil.

Use paper towels or a clean kitchen towel to pat zucchini and eggplant until dry on the surface.

Place the slices on a baking sheet lined with parchment paper. Brush olive oil on top and season with pepper.

Bake (or broil) for 15-20 minutes or until golden brown on both sides, flipping once halfway through. You can also fry the vegetables in a large skillet or cook on a grill.

When done, place on a serving platter. Drizzle olive oil and freshly-squeezed lemon juice on top.

Serve with cheese cubes, almonds, olives, yogurt, and leafy greens.

Greek low carb keftedes bowls with tzatziki

Things Needed

Tzatziki

4 oz. cucumber, grated

1 cup (6⅓ oz.) Greek yogurt (4% fat)

1 garlic clove, crushed

1 tbsp lemon juice

1 tsp lemon zest

2 tbsp olive oil

1 tbsp fresh dill, chopped

salt and pepper, to taste

Greek salad

5 oz. cucumber, sliced and halved

7 oz. cherry tomatoes, halved

3 oz. (9 tbsp) green bell peppers, sliced

1 oz. (2¾ tbsp) red onions, sliced

½ cup (2⅔ oz.) feta cheese, crumbled

1 oz. (3⅓ tbsp) olives, pitted

1 tsp dried oregano

2 tbsp olive oil

Meatballs

1 lb ground lamb

½ tsp salt

½ tsp pepper

1 oz. (2¾ tbsp) yellow onions, finely chopped

2 garlic cloves, crushed

2 tsp dried parsley

1 tsp dried oregano

1 tsp dried mint

1 large egg

½ cup (2 oz.) almond flour or 2.5 tbs coconut flour

1 tbsp ghee or butter, for greasing

Method

Tzatziki

Put the cucumber into a bowl. Add the yogurt, garlic, lemon juice, lemon zest, olive oil, and dill.

Add salt and pepper to taste. Mix until combined, then set to the side.

Greek salad

Place the cucumber, cherry tomatoes, green pepper, and red onion in a bowl.

Add the feta, olives, and oregano. Drizzle with olive oil.

Meatballs

Combine all the Ingredientsfor the meatballs in a bowl. Using your hands, form the mixture into 1" (2.5 cm) meatballs (about 33 g/1.2 oz each).

Grease a large skillet with the ghee. Once hot, add the meatballs in a single layer. Cook for about 10 minutes turning with a fork until browned on all sides and cooked through, or until the meat reaches a temperature of 160°F (71°C). Remove from the heat.

For serving

Portion the Greek salad into bowls, add meatballs, and serve with tzatziki on top.

Tips

Refrigerate the meatballs and tzatziki in separate airtight containers for up to four days.

If you want thicker tzatziki, you can squeeze out the liquid in the grated cucumber before mixing it with the other things,

Slow-cooked chicken with broccoli salad

Things Needed

5 lime leaves

1 tbsp coriander seed

1 tbsp ground ginger

½ tsp ground black pepper

1 cup (6⅓ oz.) Greek yogurt (4% fat) or other type of yogurt with a high fat content

3 lbs chicken legs

2 tsp salt

2 limes for serving (optional)

Broccoli Salad

1 lb (5 cups) broccoli

1 cup mayonnaise

½ cup (¼ oz.) chopped fresh cilantro

salt and pepper

Method

Grind the spices and mix with the yogurt. Salt the chicken and put it in a plastic bag. Pour in the yogurt marinade and massage it into the chicken.

Marinate (in the refrigerator) for 2-3 hours or overnight. If you are in a rush, marinate for at least 15 minutes at room temperature.

Put chicken and marinade in a slow cooker and cook on high heat for 2 hours or low for 3 hours. Remove and let cool. You can prepare up to this step a day ahead.

Prepare the grill and finish off the chicken with a nice browned surface, about 5-10 minutes on each side, depending on size and heat.

If you don't have access to a grill, you can sear the boiled chicken in the oven using the broiler setting. Cut the limes in half and fry or grill alongside the chicken, cut side down. They add a wonderful flavor.

Broccoli and cilantro salad

Boil the broccoli in lightly salted water; a minute or two is enough.

Mix the mayonnaise with freshly chopped cilantro and add the broccoli. Season with salt and pepper to taste.

Serve paired with the chicken, with an extra dollop of butter or mayonnaise on the side.

Tip

Can't find lime leaves? Substitute with any two of the following (per leaf): ½ bay leaf, ½ tsp lime zest, or ¼ tsp fresh lemon thyme.

Chicken skewers with low carb fries and spinach dip

Things Needed

Chicken skewers

2 lbs boneless chicken thighs, cut into 1" (2.5 cm) pieces

1 tsp salt

¼ tsp ground black pepper

2 tbsp olive oil

1 tsp garlic powder

1 tsp dried thyme

8 wooden skewers

Celery root fries

1¾ lbs celery root or rutabaga

2 tbsp olive oil

½ tsp salt

¼ tsp ground black pepper

Spinach dip

½ cup (3 oz.) Greek yogurt (4% fat)

¼ cup mayonnaise

2 oz. frozen spinach, chopped

¼ tsp ground black pepper

2 tbsp dried parsley

1 tbsp dried dill

1 tsp onion powder

½ tsp salt

2 tsp lemon juice

Method

Preheat the oven to 400°F (200°C).

Put the marinade Ingredientsin a bowl and mix.
Add the chicken. Set aside and allow to marinate
for 10–20 minutes at room temperature.

Peel the celery root. Cut into 0.5" (1 cm) thick
strips.

Place the fries on a baking sheet lined with
parchment paper. Season with salt and pepper.
Drizzle with oil and mix everything thoroughly.
Bake in the oven for 20 minutes to start with
(about 50 minutes in total or until crisp).

Thread the chicken on the skewers and spread
them out on another baking sheet lined with
parchment paper or preferably on a roasting rack.

Put them in the oven together with the fries for 20-30 minutes or until they are cooked.

To make the dip, remove the excess liquid from the thawed spinach. Add into a bowl and mix well with the other dip **Things Needed**.

Serve the chicken skewers with the celery-root fries and spinach dip. Garnish with some fresh thyme and season with salt and pepper to taste.

Ethiopian spicy doro wat soup

Things Needed

¼ cup coconut oil or lard

1 (4 oz.) yellow onion, finely chopped

1 garlic clove, minced

1 tbsp berbere seasoning

2 tsp fine sea salt

2½ lbs chicken breasts, cut into ¾" (2 cm) chunks

4 cups chicken broth

8 hard-boiled eggs

Method

Place the oil in a 6-quart Instant Pot and press Sauté. Once melted, add the onion, garlic, berbere seasoning, and salt and cook for 10 minutes or until the onion starts to caramelize. Press Cancel to stop the Sauté.

Add the chicken and broth to the instant pot. Seal the lid, press Pressure Cook or Manual, and set the timer for 20 minutes. Once finished, turn the valve to venting for a quick release.

Slice each hard-boiled egg in half. Serve the chicken and onion mixture in bowls with two egg halves in each bowl.

DELIGHTFUL RECIPES FOR SNACKS

Keto cheddar cheese and bacon balls

Things Needed

5 oz. bacon

5 oz. (⅔ cup) cream cheese

5 oz. (1¼ cups) cheddar cheese

2 oz. butter, at room temperature

½ tsp pepper (optional)

½ tsp chili flakes (optional)

Method

In a frying pan, fry the bacon until golden brown. Remove from the pan, and let cool completely on paper towels.

Crumble or chop the bacon into small pieces and place in a medium-sized bowl.

In a bigger bowl, mix the grease left over from frying the bacon with all the remaining **Ingredients**by hand, or with an electric handmixer.

Place the big bowl in the fridge for 15 minutes to set.

Make 24 walnut-sized balls, using two spoons. Roll them in the crumbled bacon and serve.

Eggplant fries

Things Needed

2¼ lbs eggplant (2 medium, globe eggplants)

2 cups (8 oz.) almond flour

1 tsp cayenne pepper (optional)

2 tsp salt

1 tsp ground black pepper

2 large eggs

2 tbsp coconut oil, melted, at room temperature

salt and ground black pepper, to taste

Method

Preheat oven to 400°F (200°C). Set aside baking sheet(s), lined with parchment paper.

Cut off the stems and peel the eggplants using a vegetable peeler or sharp knife. Cut into 3" x 1/2" (8 x 1.2 cm) French-fry pieces. Set aside.

In a shallow bowl, stir together the almond flour, cayenne pepper, salt, and black pepper. Place the eggs and coconut oil in a small bowl, and whisk together until blended.

With one hand, dip several eggplant pieces in the egg mixture, and coat on all sides. Let excess egg drip off, and then use the other hand to lightly coat each piece in the flour mixture. Transfer to the baking sheet(s) and repeat until done. (see Tip)

Place on the middle oven rack and bake for 7 - 8 minutes, turn fries over, and bake for another 7 - 8 minutes, until crispy and golden brown.

Salad sandwiches

Things Needed

2 oz. (1¼ cups) Romaine lettuce or baby gem lettuce

2 tbsp mayonnaise

1 oz. (4 tbsp) edam cheese or other cheese of your liking

½ (3½ oz.) avocado, sliced

4 (2½ oz.) cherry tomatoes, sliced

Method

Rinse the lettuce thoroughly and use it as a base for the toppings.

Spread butter or mayonnaise on the lettuce leaves, and layer the cheese, avocado, and tomato on top. Enjoy!

Keto sandwich with smoked salmon and horseradish cream

Things Needed

7 oz. smoked salmon

½ cup mayonnaise or sour cream

1 oz. fresh horseradish, grated

Mug bread

2 tbsp almond flour

2 tbsp coconut flour

1½ tsp baking powder

¼ tsp salt

2 eggs

2 tbsp heavy whipping cream

1 tsp butter

Serving

2 tbsp butter

½ oz. (⅔ cup) arugula lettuce

¼ (1¾ oz.) small zucchini, finely sliced (optional)

1 tbsp pink peppercorns (optional)

Method

Chop the salmon into small pieces and mix with mayonnaise and freshly grated horseradish. Set aside in the refrigerator until it's time to serve.

Mix together all dry Ingredientsfor the bread. Crack in the egg and stir in the cream. Combine until smooth. Pour into well-greased mugs or glass molds. 1 egg equals one portion / mug.

Microwave on high (approximately 700 watts) for 2 minutes. Check if the bread is done in the middle – if not, microwave for another 15-30 seconds.

Let cool and remove from the mug. Slice in half and toast for best taste and texture.

Spread butter on each slice, add lettuce leaves, thinly sliced zucchini and a generous dollop of the salmon and horseradish cream. Top with crushed pink peppercorns.

Edamame crisps

Things Needed

6 oz. (1 cup) edamame beans

1 tsp olive oil

¼ tsp salt

½ tsp paprika powder

2½ oz. freshly grated Parmesan cheese

2 tbsp sunflower seeds

Method

Preheat the oven to 400°F (200°C). Line a baking tray with parchment paper.

Rinse and pat the edamame beans dry, drizzle with olive oil and sprinkle over salt and paprika powder. Spread the edamame out on the baking tray. Bake for 10 minutes.

Meanwhile, finely grate the Parmesan cheese.

When the edamame have baked for 10 minutes, remove them from the oven. Move the edamame closer together, so they're almost touching each other. Sprinkle over the sunflower seeds and heap the grated Parmesan on top. Spread out the Parmesan so that all the edamame are covered.

Return the tray to the oven for another 8-10 minutes until the Parmesan has melted.

Allow to cool and crisp up. Break into pieces and serve.

Low carb banana bread

Things Needed

2 (7 oz.) very ripe bananas, cut in smaller pieces

6 large eggs

6 tbsp butter melted

2 tsp vanilla extract

3 cups (12 oz.) almond flour

4 tsp ground cinnamon

2 tsp baking powder

⅛ tsp salt

Method

Preheat the oven to 350°F (180°C).

Add the banana, eggs, vanilla, and melted butter to a food processor or a medium-sized bowl if you are using an electric hand mixer. Mix until smooth.

Add the dry **Ingredients**and mix until well-combined.

Line a loaf pan 9" x 5" (23 x 13 cm) with parchment paper and fill with the batter.

Bake in the oven for 50 minutes or until you insert a knife and it comes out clean. Check the loaf halfway through. If the top is getting too brown, cover loosely with tin foil.

Let cool on the rack for at least 30 minutes. Cut in slices and enjoy with butter or low-carb nut butter.

Low carb cream cheese with herbs

Things Needed

8 oz. (1 cup) cream cheese

2 tsp olive oil

½ cup (¼ oz.) fresh parsley or fresh basil, chopped

1 garlic clove, minced

1 tsp lemon zest

salt and pepper, to taste

4 (5⅔ oz.) celery stalks, or other fresh vegetables of your liking

Method

Stir all Ingredientsinto the cream cheese. Let sit in the refrigerator for at least 10 minutes to let all the flavors develop. Add salt if needed.

Rinse celery stalks, cut into 2-3 inch lengths, and serve together with the soft cheese.

Keto French toast

Things Needed

Mug bread

1 tsp butter

2 tbsp almond flour

2 tbsp coconut flour

1½ tsp baking powder

1 pinch salt

2 large eggs

2 tbsp heavy whipping cream

Batter

2 large eggs

2 tbsp heavy whipping cream

½ tsp ground cinnamon

1 pinch salt

2 tbsp butter

Method

Grease a large mug or glass dish with a flat bottom
with butter.

Mix together all dry Ingredientsin the mug with a fork or spoon. Crack in the egg and stir in the cream. Combine until smooth and make sure there are no lumps.

Microwave on high (approximately 700 watts) for 2 minutes. Check if the bread is done in the middle – if not, microwave for another 15-30 seconds.

Let cool and remove from the mug. Slice in half.

In a bowl or deep plate, whisk together the eggs, cream and cinnamon with a pinch of salt. Pour over the bread slices and let them get soaked. Turn them around a few times so the bread slices absorb as much of the egg mixture as possible.

Fry in plenty of butter and serve immediately.

Low carb pumpkin spice crackers

Things Needed

⅓ cup (1¼ oz.) coconut flour

2 tbsp pumpkin pie spice

¾ cup (3⅔ oz.) sunflower seeds

¾ cup (4½ oz.) flaxseed

⅓ cup (1⅔ oz.) sesame seeds

1 tbsp ground psyllium husk powder

1 tsp salt

3 tbsp coconut oil, melted

1⅓ cups water

Method

Preheat the oven to 300°F (150°C). Mix together all dry Things Needed.

Stir and add water and oil. Stir well and let sit for 2–3 minutes.

Spread out on a baking sheet lined with parchment paper and place in the middle of the oven. Bake for 30 minutes. Use a timer to keep track of time.

Check the crackers. Bake for another 30 minutes and perhaps lower the heat towards the end.

Make sure the crackers are dry. If not, let dry some more. Crack into pieces when cooled down. Keep in a tight-fitting container.

8

TO WRAP THINGS UP!

The Hollywood Diet offers a realistic and effective way to lose weight and live healthier. By emphasizing portion control, balanced nutrition, and fresh, whole foods, this diet helps you make sustainable changes to your eating habits. It might seem challenging at first, but the Hollywood Diet promotes a mindful way of eating that can bring lasting results.

One of the great things about the Hollywood Diet is its flexibility. It allows for occasional treats, making it easier to stick with your goals even during social events and special occasions. This balance helps you weave healthy eating into your everyday life without feeling like you're missing out. The focus on healthy choices helps you build a positive relationship with food, supporting long-term wellness beyond just shedding pounds.

In the end, the Hollywood Diet is more than a quick fix—it's a path to a healthier, more energetic life. By embracing its principles, you can achieve your fitness goals, boost your energy, and improve your overall well-being. Remember, it's about being consistent and patient. The Hollywood Diet is not just about reaching your goal; it's about enjoying the journey to becoming the best version of yourself.

9 798327 901193